Weight loss
How to lose weight and stay slim with Homeopathy and Schuessler salts (cell salts)

Robert Kopf

Copyright © 2023 Robert Kopf

All rights reserved

ISBN 9798481115191

CONTENT

Introduction

Metabolic blockages in the treatment of weight gain and overweight   page 10

Weight Loss - Lose weight and stay slim with Homeopathy   page 13

Lose weight and stay slim with Schuessler salts   page 74

Epilogue   page 99

INTRODUCTION

Robert Kopf, Author of Naturopathy and Traditional healer

Translated from german edition by the author

The metabolic activity decides about our figure. It determines whether we stay lean even though we eat and drink according to our mood, or whether we become fat, even if we eat like a sparrow.

If you gain weight, you're more likely to develop a number of potentially serious health problems like diabetes, high cholesterol, high blood pressure, metabolic disorders, heart disease, stroke, cancer and osteoarthritis.

Causes of weight gain and overweight are hormonal imbalance, metabolic disorders, a sluggish liver activity, disturbances of bowel function, lack of exercise, inadequate fat burning, heredity, an underactive thyroid, social and economic problems, overeating with food that contains too much fat, salt, sugar, flavor enhancers and sweeteners.

In the homeopathic and biochemical treatment (Schuessler salts) of weight gain and overweight, detoxification therapies serve the activation of metabolism, the immune system and strengthening the body's circulation and connective tissue. It cleans, de-acidifies the body, is mineralizing and leads to a balanced life energy.

Weight gain and overweight can be caused and reinforced by a mineral deficiency and an acidification of the body. Mineral deficiency and acidification in turn weaken the hormonal system, connective tissue and immune system.

Also a defective metabolism favors weight gain and overweight, chronic health problems and is often the result of a disturbance of mineral intake and mineral distribution.

Although we may receive enough minerals in our food, in the event of a metabolic disorder, not all of the minerals may reach the cells.

The use of homeopathic remedies and Schuessler salts is a good way to compensate this mineral deficiency in a natural way and to treat weight gain and overweight.

Stress as well as environmental toxins hinder the mineral transport through the cell membranes. This is where the effect of Homeopathy and Schuessler salts works. They activate the excretion of toxins and acids. The basal metabolic rate increases and the self-healing power of the body is activated.

First I like to explain you the therapies for the treatment and prevention of weight gain and overweight offered in this guide:

Homeopathy was developed about 200 years ago by Samuel Hahnemann. The three basic principles of Homeopathy are the simile rule, homeopathic drug testing and detection of individual disease.

The most important principle is the principle of Similarity (simile rule), which was formulated in 1796 by Hahnemann.

It states that a patient should be treated with the remedy, which can cause in its original state similar symptoms in healthy people like the existing disease. It notes primarily the main complaints of the patient.

Together with a few differentiating additional informations (modalities) then the right remedy will be found for the treatment of weight gain and overweight.

The dosage depends on the condition of the patient. As the patient improves, the distances between the medication will be gradually extended.

What happens if you choose the wrong remedy? Nothing - just as a key does not turn in the wrong door lock, a wrong homeopathic remedy does not cause any reaction in the body.

The homeopathic remedies are available as D-, C- and LM potencies.

For the beginners in Homeopathy, I recommend the use of lower D-potencies. Higher potencies (D200, C and LM potencies) should only be given by an expert, as they go very deep in their effects and are often used only once.

Schuessler salts (also named homeopathic cell salts, tissue salts, Biochemistry) for the treatment and prevention of weight gain and overweight

In the 19th Century the german physician Dr. Wilhelm Heinrich Schuessler (1821 to 1898) developed his health cure with homeopathic mineral salts. In recent years this therapy celebrated a comeback.

In his studies Schuessler discovered twelve mineral compounds, comprised each of a base and an acid, which play a crucial role in the function and structure of the body.

He developed his own system with which many diseases can be treated in a natural way (also weight gain and overweight).

Schuessler focused his search on mineral salts and trace elements, which are found in every cell of the body and called his method of healing "Biochemistry" (chemistry of life).

It is based on the assumption that nearly every disease is caused because of the lack of a specific mineral salt. This leads to dysregulations inside the cells. The molecules cannot flow freely.

A mineral salt deficiency arises from the fact that the cells cannot optimally use the minerals. To improve their absorption, mineral salts therefore have to be highly diluted (potentized). Schuessler used the homeopathic potencies D3 (3x), D6 (6x) and D12 (12x) for his therapy. In general, the 6x (dilution 1:1 million) or 12x (1:1 trillion) is taken.

In this homeopathic and naturopathic adviser, I will give you recommendations how to treat and prevent weight gain and overweight naturally with Homeopathy, herbal tinctures and Schuessler salts (also named homeopathic cell salts, tissue salts).

I will present you the most proven homeopathic remedies and Schuessler salts, including the appropriate potency and dosage.

Naturopathy works holistically. It does not treat single symptoms only. It treats the whole body, mind and soul.

I wish you much success, joy in life and especially your health.

Robert Kopf

Metabolic blockages in the treatment of weight gain and overweight

There are several metabolic blockages which you have to treat for to deacidify and detoxify the body of people suffering from weight gain and overweight.

Metabolic blockage No. 1: The acid-base balance

Too much sugar, white flour, meat and sausage acidifies the body. In order to neutralize the acids precious bases are consumed. What is not neutralized, ends up as a "hazardous waste" in the connective tissue and leads to its acidity.

The metabolic process slows down. We gain weight despite calorie conscious diet and exercise.

Metabolic blockage No. 2: The connective tissue

The connective tissue is more than just a connection between the organs. It serves as a nutrient storage and intermediate storage of metabolic products. In the connective tissue the cells dispose their waste products. That the toxins can leave the body, enough mineral salts must be present.

A mineral deficiency causes metabolic residues, acidification and overload with toxins. They remain in the connective tissue and bind water. It comes to overweight and water retention (edema) in the tissues of the body.

Metabolic blockage No. 3: The digestion

Environmental pollution, lush diet and medication burden the liver, our central metabolic organ. Stomach, pancreas and intestines suffer with.

Many metabolic processes stalled and it comes to weight gain, constipation, bloating and stomach problems.

Metabolic blockage No. 4: Our water Resources

Every day the organism produces acids and waste products that have to be filtered out by the kidneys. But part of it also ends up in the connective tissue, because for the removal mineral salts are absent. We gain weight.

Metabolic blockage No. 5: The protein digestion

Protein is essential for the production of enzymes, hormones, muscles and the connective tissue. However, in the cleavage of proteins ammonia is formed (a strong cytotoxin). The liver converts the ammonia into non-toxic urea, which is excreted in the urine.

Therefore, a high intake of protein is a strong decontamination work for the liver and our two kidneys. The result is overweight.

Metabolic blockage No. 6: The digestion of fat

We need fats because they provide essential fatty acids. But fat is also the best energy storage in times of need. The body hoards it especially in the thighs and hips, the abdomen and buttocks.

But the adipose tissue is also a deposit for toxins. This forces weight gain.

Metabolic blockage No. 7: The carbohydrate digestion

Carbohydrates are energy pure. But in abundance they are also responsible for weight gain and acidification of the body. What is not burned, will be converted and stored in fat.

Especially sweets and white flour products are dangerous. They let the blood sugar level rise up rapidly. This leads to a strong insulin release.

Insulin normalizes blood sugar. At the same time burning fat is broken. Insulin leads fats from the meal into the fat stores of the body. In addition, it holds back water in the body and causes rapidly new hunger.

More information for the treatment of your metabolism you will find in my book:

Metabolism, Metabolic syndrome - Treatment with Homeopathy and Schuessler salts

Weight Loss - Lose weight and stay slim with Homeopathy

Now I will give you recommendations how to find back to a normal weight with the help of Homeopathy and to activate your metabolism.

In addition to your homeopathic treatment, you may make a de-acidification health cure of your body with the following recipe:

320 grams of Sodium bicarbonate (Natrium hydrogenkarbonat)
50 grams of Potassium hydrogen carbonate (Kalium hydrogencarbonat)
70 grams of Calcium citrate (Calciumcitrat)
40 grams of Calcium phosphate (Calciumphosphat)
20 grams of Magnesium citrate (Magnesiumcitrat)
Dissolve 1 teaspoon in 250 ml of lukewarm water daily at 10 am and 4 pm and drink in small sips.

During the day time, in addition to your homeopathic treatment, drink 3 cups of tea for the kidneys. In the evening drink one cup of tea for the liver. This will clean the blood and connective tissue and the toxins, acids and metabolic waste products will be excreted quickly.

1) Liver support tea and detoxing the body:

Semen Cardui marianae 50.0 (milk thistle), Rhizoma Tormentillae 15.0 (bloodroot), Radix cum Herba Taraxaci 30.0 (dandelion root and herb), Fructi anisidine (anise) 20.0, Fructi Foeniculi (fennel) 20.0, Folia crispae mentha (mint) 15.0
Mix the above listed items together. Add 1 tablespoon into 1 cup (250 ml) cold water and cover for 8 hours. Cook 3 minutes. Let sit covered for 10 minutes and then strain. Drink 1 cup in the evening.

2) Tea for the kidneys and the excretion of metabolic waste and acids through the urinary tract:

Folia Betulae (birch leaves) 30.0, Herba urticae (nettle herb) 30.0, Herba Equiseti (horsetail) 20.0, Herba Virgaureae (goldenrod) 20.0
Mix the above listed ingredients together. Add 2 teaspoons into 1 cup (250 ml) of hot water, let sit covered for 10 minutes. Strain to drink. Drink 3 cups daily.

3) If you suffer from allergies (often a cause of overweight), alternate daily the 2 above mentioned teas with a tea for the treatment of allergies to sensitize the body for the treatment with the Schuessler salts and Homeopathy:

Radix Imperatoriae 20 g, Radix Pimpinellae 20 g, Herba Euphrasiae 10 g, Herba Rutae hortensis 30 g, Rhizoma Graminis 10 g, Herba Absinthii 10 g
Mix the above listed ingredients together. Add 1 teaspoon into 1 cup (250 ml) of water, cook 2 minutes, let sit covered for 10 minutes. Strain to drink. Drink 3 cups daily.

Pay attention to an adequate hydration (water, tea, unsweetened juices).

The kidneys can only extract metabolic waste products if there is enough liquid available. If you exercise a lot, you need more fluid. The water supports the elimination of toxins and waste products of the metabolism. In addition, it prevents hunger.

Drink the most until the afternoon. In the evening drink as little as possible to relieve the bladder.

For enhancing the effect of the homeopathic medicine dissolve the globules in a small glas of water and drink in small sips. Swallow after 1 minute. For stirring please do not use metal spoon.

Do not count the globules in the hand. The manual welding destroys the sprayed drug.

Avoid during the homeopathic treatment the consumption of nicotine, alcohol and spicy foods. They reduce the effectiveness of the sensitive homeopathic remedies.

Abrotanum 3x
Increases during the treatment of overweight the blood flow to the digestive organs.
Opens the small arteries and veins (capillaries). As a result, the metabolism is stimulated.
Strenghtens the connective tissue and the immune system.
Circulatory disorders of the brain.
Increases blood circulation of the brain.
High blood pressure
Rheumatism alternates with hemorrhoids.
Sharp urine
Kidney and bladder diseases.
3 times a day, take 10 globules, let them melt in your mouth.

Absinthium tincture
The basic remedy for the treatment of overweight due to stomach and liver weakness.
Strengthens the spleen (important for the treatment of obesity)
Strengthen the immune system, extracts environmental toxins and resolves metabolic blockages.
Gastritis and stomach diseases.
Strengthens the stomach.
Stimulates the function of the pancreas.
Promotes the formation of bile - the intestine is stimulated by it (70% of our immune system are located in the intestine). Intestines healthy, man healthy!
Absinthium is a basic remedy for the treatment of diseases of the digestive organs.
Bloating
3 times a day, add 15 drops in some water and drink in small sips.

Acidum hydrofluoricum 12x
Overweight
Strengthens the connective tissue in the treatment of too much body weight and prevents wrinkling of the skin.
Strengthens the blood vessels.
2 times a day, take 5 globules, let them melt in your mouth.

Acidum muriaticum 4x
Overweight
Connective tissue weakness
Anemia and iron deficiency
Acidum muriaticum enhances the absorption of iron in the small intestine.
3 times a day, take 10 globules, let them melt in your mouth.

Acidum nitricum 6x

Overweight due to mental stress, neurasthenia and overwrought senses.
Heart problems and insomnia.
Acid regurgitation, sour and bitter taste after eating.
Gastritis and peptic ulcer.
The person has a cold quickly.
Strong smelling urine.
Acidum nitricum strengthens the immune system, nerves and energy.
The "Acidum nitricum-Type":
The face is dark and looks dried out.
The patient asks for salty and fatty foods.
Life weariness, hopelessness, rejects consolation.
3 times a day, take 5 globules, let them melt in your mouth.

Acidum phosphoricum 3x

An important metabolic remedy for the treatment overweight.
Normalizes the metabolism and excretes metabolic blockages.
Strengthens the pancreas and the connective tissue of the intestines.
Acidum phosphoricum strengthen the nerves and immune system.
The patient is tired and weak.
Loss of concentration, dizziness.
Needs rest and warmth.
3 times a day, take 10 globules, let them melt in your mouth.

Acidum sulph 6x (Acidum sulfuricum D6)
Overweight due to hormonal changes.
Depression, nervousness and anxiety.
Heart problems and sleep disorders
Vomiting, nausea and sweating
Diarrhea and bloating
Very helpful for the treatment of stomach diseases and a weakened immune system.
The symptoms are worse at night, in movement and touch.
3 times a day, take 5 globules, let them melt in your mouth.

Adonis vernalis tincture
Overweight due to cardiac insufficiency.
Low blood pressure
Adonis vernalis invigorates the heart.
3 times a day, add 15 drops in some water and drink in small sips.

Aesculus tincture
Overweight
Venous circulatory disorders
Strengthens the veins
Venous congestion
Extracts edema
3 times a day, add 15 drops in some water and drink in small sips.

Aethiops antimonialis 6x
Overweight
Eczema and dermatitis with blistering of the skin.
Frequent skin rash
Allergy with swollen eyelids
Severe photophobia
3 times a day, take 5 globules, let them melt in your mouth.

Agnus castus 3x
Overweight and immunodeficiency of women in menopause.
Menopausal symptoms
Weather sensitivity, mood swings and depression of women in menopause.
Agnus castus has a regulating effect on the female hormonal system.
3 times a day, take 10 globules, let them melt in your mouth.

Agrimonia eupatoria 3x
Overweight
Forces blood flow to the digestive organs.
Stimulates digestion, metabolism and the immune system.
Strengthens the stomach, liver, pancreas and intestine (more then 70% of our immune system are located in the intestine).
Edema due to a liver weakness.
Bloating
Agrimonia promotes the formation of urea and the extraction of toxins.
Proven in ascites.
Helps to strengthen the defense.
Purifies and detoxifies the body.
3 times a day, take 10 globules, let them melt in your mouth.

Ambra 30x

Overweight of people with nervous exhaustion.
Circulatory problems, meteorosensitivity and hypersensitivity.
Depressed mood and vegetative disturbances.
Nervousness and nervous exhaustion due to worries.
Dysregulation of the autonomic nervous system.
Can not unwind in the evening.
The person don`t like many people around, gets easily upset.
The "Amber" type:
The person is unstable, restless and weak.
Blushes easily
Vascular calcification
In the morning take 5 globules. Let them melt in your mouth.

Ammi visnaga tincture

Overweight
Connective tissue weakness
Low blood pressure due to a weak heart.
Ammi visnaga relaxes the bronchial tubes and the coronary arteries. Thus, the body cells are better supplied with oxygen and nutrients.
Chest tightness and angina pectoris.
Circulatory disorders of the heart.
Stimulates blood flow to the heart.
3 times a day, add 15 drops in a small glass of water and drink in small sips.

Ammonium carb. 12x (Ammonium carbonicum D12)
Overweight
Depression, high blood pressure and immunodeficiency of thick women, panting and gasping for air.
The patient is restless, fearful, angry and short of breath.
The person promises much, but does nothing.
Watery and red eyes.
Prone Skin
Worsening of the symtoms at night.
2 times a day, take 5 globules, let them melt in your mouth.

Angelica tincture
Overweight
To strengthen the digestive system and metabolism.
Strengthens blood circulation and the immune system. The majority of our immune system is located in the abdomen.
Gastritis and stomach diseases.
Calms the entire abdomen.
Diabetes
Weakness of the digestive organs.
Stimulates the blood flow to stomach, pancreas and liver and normalizes the function of the digestive organs.
Intestines healthy, man healthy!
3 times a day, add 15 drops in some water and drink in small sips.

Antimony crudum 4x (Antimonium crudum D4)

Overweight

Connective tissue weakness

Gastritis and indigestion

Nausea and vomiting

Thick and milky white coating on the tongue.

Diarrhea and constipation alternate.

Itchy skin

3 times a day, take 10 globules, let them melt in your mouth.

Apium graveolens tincture

Too much body weight and edema.

Extracts edema out of the body.

3 times a day, add 15 drops in a small glass of water and drink in small sips.

Apocynum cannabinum 3x

Overweight with edema due to a weakness of the heart and kidneys.

Stimulates the heart and kidneys.

Stimulates the elimination of edema.

3 times a day, take 10 globules, let them melt in your mouth.

Argentum nitricum 6x (Silver nitrate D6)
Overweight
Connective tissue weakness
For the treatment of people who are prone to swollen glands, rashes and chronic diseases.
Too much stomach acid
Also an excellent remedy for the treatment of stomach ulcers.
The face is dark and has a dried-up appearance.
The person is always in a hurry, hectic and restless.
He believes the time passes by too slowly.
The "silver nitrate patient" demands for sweets and sugar but he can not tolerate.
He also like to have salt and cool fresh air.
The patient suffers from anxiety, haste and bloating.
Argentum nitricum strengthens the immune system.
The person catch quickly a cold.
Sometimes the complaints start with sunrise and stops with sunset.
3 times a day, take 5 globules, let them melt in your mouth.

Arnica 3x

Overweight

Connective tissue weakness

Diseases of the arteries and veins.

Promotes healing processes, blood circulation and strengthens the blood vessels.

Arnica is the main remedy for arterial and venous circulatory disorders. As a result, the body is better supplied with oxygen and nutrients and the metabolism will be strengthened.

The Arnica patient perceives his body sore and bruised, the bed is too hard.

The patient is afraid of contact with other people.

A strange symptom: He pretends to be healthy, even if he is sick.

3 times a day, take 10 globules, let them melt in your mouth.

Arsenicum album 6x

Overweight
Connective tissue weakness
The skin is waxy, dry and flaky.
Cold, dull and blemished skin.
Nervous itching
Eczema, boils, lichen, carbuncles, gangrene, shallow ulcers.
The secretions are corrosive, excoriating, watery and burning.
Worse by cold air
Frequent colds
Desire for fresh air, despite feeling cold.
Great restlessness, anxiety and fatigue.
Want always to move.
The person is sensitive to cold, choosy and frightened.
A broken and emaciated person with a weak immune system.
Polyuria (frequent urination with a lot of urine).
Great thirst
Melancholy, despair, indifference, depression and anxiety.
The person is exhausted, pale, emaciated, frightened and tired of life.
Fear of death and sorrow.
Aggravation of his symptoms at midnight. His worst time is between 12 clock at night and 2 clock in the morning (2 am).
The abdomen is sensitive to pressure.
Circulatory problems
Sunken face with hollow eyes.
3 times a day, take 5 globules, let them melt in your mouth.

Aurum chloratum 6x

Overweight

Eliminates metabolic blockages during the treatment of overweight.

Supports weight loss

Increases well-being

3 times a day, take 5 globules, let them melt in your mouth.

Aurum iodatum 6x (Aurum jodatum D6)

Overweight of persons with high blood pressure and red face.

Sclerosis of the brain.

The person will be increasingly depressed, irritable and jaded.

Decline in memory

A grumpy patient

The main symptoms:

Worries about the future even if he's okay.

Always takes everything very seriously.

The accompanying symptom: Great sensitivity to cold.

3 times a day, take 5 globules, let them melt in your mouth.

Aurum metallicum 12x
Overweight caused by metabolic blockade.
Red-cheeked and obese people.
Suppuration and inflammation of the skin.
Aurum metallicum eliminates metabolic blockages and strengthens the immune system.
Induration of glandular organs.
The main remedy for all venous problems.
High blood pressure and red face.
An obese person with dimpled skin, immunodeficiency, cardiac insufficiency and angina pectoris.
Sclerosis of the brain.
The person will be increasingly depressed, irritable and jaded.
Decline in memory
A grumpy patient
Hopeless blackness. He talks about death.
Worries about the future, even if he's okay.
Always takes everything very seriously.
The accompanying symptom: Great sensitivity to cold.
2 times a day, take 5 globules, let them melt in the mouth.

Barium iodatum 6x (Barium jodatum D6)
Overweight because of an underactive thyroid gland (causes a slow metabolism).
Barium iodatum strengthens the thyroid. This stimulates the metabolism and increases the body temperature. This in turn strengthens the immune system.
High blood pressure due to arteriosclerosis.
Stimulates the brain metabolism.
Strengthens the immune system.
Stimulates the arterial blood flow too. Thus, the body cells are better supplied with oxygen and nutrients.
3 times a day, take 5 globules, let them melt in your mouth.

Berberis 3x
Overweight
Supports the function of the liver and pancreas.
Diseases of the liver and gallbladder.
Diabetes
3 times a day, take 10 globules, let it melt in the mouth.

Bursa pastoris tincture
Overweight and edema
Strengthens the blood vessels.
3 times a day, add 15 drops in some water and drink in small sips.

Calabar 6x
Overweight
Strengthens the metabolism of liver and pancreas for to lose weight.
Stimulates digestion and metabolism of the body.
3 times a day, take 5 globules, let them melt in your mouth.

Calcium carbonicum 12x (Calcarea 12x)

Overweight with neurasthenia, nervous weakness and depression.
Old and obstinate constipation, persistent bloating.
Regurgitation and vomiting.
The patient is gloomy, moody and indifferent.
An important remedy of "lymphatic constitution" for the treatment of too much body weight, depression, weakness, immune deficiency and slow metabolism.
Rashes and frequent colds.
Sour sweat after the slightest exertion on the head and neck.
Strong foot perspiration
A fearful and hesitant person.
Aggravation of symptoms by cold and damp weather, during full moon.
Improvement by heat and drought.
2 times a day, take 5 globules, let them melt in your mouth.

Calcium sulph 6x (Calcium sulfuricum D6)

Overweight
Connective tissue weakness
Skin diseases with ulcerations of the skin and subcutaneous tissue.
Strengthens the immune system.
3 times a day, take 5 globules, let them melt in your mouth.

Calendula tincture
Overweight
To deacidify and detoxify the body.
Purifies the blood.
Strengthens the lymphatic system (important for a strong metabolism).
Increases the metabolic function.
Invigorating the blood vessels and lymph vessels.
An excellent wound healing remedy.
Eliminates inflammations
3 times a day, add 15 drops in a small glass of water and drink in small sips.

Capsicum 6x
Overweight
Has a warming effect and stimulates the metabolism.
Capsicum dissolves fat deposits.
General chilliness
Burning of the skin and mucous membranes.
For the treatment of mucous membranes and gastrointestinal tract.
3 times a day, take 5 globules, let them melt in your mouth.

Cardui benedikti 3x
Overweight
Strengthens pancreas and liver.
Edema due to liver insufficiency.
Stimulates bile flow.
Bloating
3 times a day, take 10 globules, let them melt in your mouth.

Carduus marianus tincture
Overweight due to liver and gall bladder diseases.
Strengthens the pancreas and liver.
Supports the metabolism of pancreas and liver.
3 times a day, add 15 drops in a small glass of water and drink in small sips.

Centaurium tincture
Overweight due to a weakness of the digestive organs.
Anemia and iron deficiency
Promotes the formation of blood
Contains iron
Strengthens the spleen (important for the treatment of anemia).
Promotes iron absorption in the small intestine.
3 times a day, add 15 drops in a small glass of water and drink in small sips.

Ceonothus 3x
If overweight is related to the spleen, for example after splenectomy or disease of the spleen.
Weight gain after gonorrhea.
The patient can not lay on his left side.
Dirty and yellowish coated tongue.
Anemia
3 times a day, take 10 globules, let them melt in your mouth.

Chelidonium 6x

Overweight with itching due to liver and gall bladder diseases.
Constant and dull pain under the inner angle of the left scapula.
Strengthens the function of pancreatic tissue and liver.
Relaxes the bile ducts.
Chelidonium excretes metabolic waste.
3 times a day, take 5 globules, let them melt in your mouth.

China 6x

Overweight due to a weakness of pancreas and liver.
China strengthens the metabolism, immune system, pancreas and liver.
Bitter taste, yellowish coated tongue.
Abdominal pressure, bloating, diarrhea, nausea and vomiting.
Frequent common colds and attacks of fever.
Modalities:
Periodic pain at certain times of day.
Improvement by firm pressure and fresh air.
Accompanying symptom: Painful hair
Circulatory problems, meteorosensitivity and neurasthenia.
Anemia
Insomnia due to flood of thoughts. General fatigue and exhaustion.
Physical and emotional hypersensitivity.
General weakness and debility.
He does not tolerate fruit or milk.
Worsening of symptoms with a light touch, drafts, cold and after the loss of body fluids.
The person is never really healthy. Subfebrile body temperature (mild fever, often after antibiotic treatment).
3 times a day, take 5 globules, let them melt in your mouth.

Cholesterinum 6x
Overweight and elevated cholesterol levels.
Pancreas- and liver disease.
Strengthens the pancreas, the liver and stimulates bile production.
Bloating
Sometimes occurs right side burning abdominal pain.
3 times a day, take 5 globules, let them melt in your mouth.

Cichorium tincture
Overweight
Strengthens liver and pancreas.
Promotes bile formation to reduce cholesterol levels.
Diabetes
3 times a day, add 15 drops in a small glass of water and drink in small sips.

Cimicifuga 12x
Overweight of women due to hormonal imbalances and in menopause.
Cimicifuga regulates the hormonal balance.
Defense weakness of women due to hormonal imbalance.
Depression, nervous agitation, insomnia and anxiety.
Pain in the abdomen and chest.
Spurious heart pain (the heart is healthy despite complaints).
Hot flashes, nervous agitation.
Depression and insomnia.
Restlessness, fear, hysteria and delusions.
A mistrustful person.
2 times a day, take 5 globules, let them melt in your mouth.

Colchicum 6x

Overweight
Connective tissue weakness
Gout and rheumatism
Joint pain
Modalities:
Worse by cold, before and during a change of weather, wet conditions, at night, from sunset to sunrise.
Worse are the symptoms also due to food smells and touch.
Improvement by heat and bed rest.
Associated symptoms:
Vibration of the muscles
Edematous swelling of the affected body region.
Twitches and spasms
The pain:
Tearing and wandering around.
Rheumatic pain especially on the left side of the body.
Keynotes:
General fatigue, inner cold
Vomiting and nausea due to food odors.
3 times a day, take 5 globules. Let them melt in your mouth.

Condurango tincture
Overweight
Weight gain due to liver weakness.
Stimulates the liver, pancreas and digestive glands.
3 times a day, add 15 drops in a small glass of water and drink in small sips.

Convallaria tincture
Overweight
Weight gain due to heart failure.
Convallaria strengthens the heart.
Low blood pressure
Cardiac insufficiency
Arrhythmia
3 times a day, add 15 drops in some water or in tea from hawthorn (Crataegus). Drink in small sips.

Crataegus tincture (hawthorn)
Overweight due to cardiac insufficiency.
Disturbance of blood pressure
Arrhythmias and angina pectoris
Circulatory problems and nervous heart
Promotes blood circulation of the heart
A perfect remedy for heart care - Crataegus prevents calcification of the coronary vessels.
3 times a day, add 15 drops in a small glass of water or in tea from the herbs of hawthorn (Crataegus). Drink in small sips.

Cynara scolymus tincture (artichoke)
Overweight
Weight gain due to an insufficient pancreas- and liver function.
Stimulates the pancreas, liver and gall bladder system.
Strengthens the liver and assists in detoxification.
An excellent protection for liver and pancreas.
3 times a day, add 15 drops in a small glass of water and drink in small sips.

Dolichos pruriens 3x
Overweight due to a liver disease.
Itching skin diseases caused by liver disease.
3 times a day, take 10 globules, let them melt in your mouth.

Equisetum tincture
Overweight
An excellent remedy for the excretion of edema.
Equisetum purifies the urinary tract.
Strengthens blood vessels and connective tissue.
Contains silica (important for the treatment of overweight)
3 times a day, add 15 drops in a small glass of water and drink in small sips.

Fel tauri 6x
Overweight with high cholesterol and hyperlipidemia.
Promotes bile formation to reduce cholesterol levels.
Promotes bile formation and thereby stimulates the disturbed fat digestion.
Strengthens liver, gallbladder and pancreas.
Bloating due to hepatobiliary disorders.
3 times a day, take 5 globules, let them melt in the mouth.

Ferrum carbonica 6x (Ferrum carbonicum D6)
Overweight
Connective tissue weakness
Anemia
Neurasthenia
Circulatory disturbances with dizziness.
Dizziness
3 times a day, take 5 globules, let them melt in your mouth.

Ferrum citricum 4x
Overweight
Connective tissue weakness
Anemia and iron deficiency
3 times a day, take 10 globules, let them melt in your mouth.

Flor de Piedra 3x
Overweight
Strengthens pancreas and liver
Assists in detoxification.
3 times a day, take 10 globules, let them melt in the mouth.

Fucus vesiculosus tincture
Overweight
Weight gain due to a weak thyroid and weak metabolism.
Stimulates the thyroid gland, metabolism and digestion.
Do not take if an overactive thyroid.
3 times a day, add 15 drops in a small glass of water and drink in small sips.

Fumaria tincture
Overweight due to a weak metabolism.
Stimulates the whole metabolism of the body.
Weak liver
3 times a day, add 15 drops in a small glass of water. Drink in small sips.

Gentiana tincture
Overweight
Connective tissue weakness
Anemia and iron deficiency
Strengthens the digestive organs.
Promotes the formation of blood.
Contains iron
Strengthens the spleen (important for the treatment of connective tissue weakness).
Promotes iron absorption in the small intestine.
3 times a day, add 15 drops in a small glass of water and drink in small sips.

Ginkgo biloba tincture
Overweight
Connective tissue weakness
Arterial circulatory disorders
Supports arterial blood flow, thereby the metabolism increases.
Stimulates blood circulation of the body and improves the oxygen uptake of the cells.
3 times a day, add 15 drops in a small glass of water and drink in small sips.

Glechoma hederacea tincture
Overweight
Anemia and iron deficiency
Promotes the formation of blood.
Contains iron
Strengthens the spleen (important for the treatment of anemia)
Promotes iron absorption in the small intestine.
3 times a day, add 15 drops in a small glass of water and drink in small sips.

Graphites 6x
Overweight
A proven homeopathic remedy for the treatment of metabolic disorders and to treat overweight.
Helps people with a slow metabolism.
Tendency to skin problems and eczema.
The skin is itchy, mostly dry, scabby, yellow and pale.
Blackheads, acne
Terrible foot sweat
Smelly night sweats
Intestinal disorders
3 times a day, take 5 globules, let them melt in the mouth.

Hamamelis virginica tincture
Overweight
Connective tissue weakness
Venous congestions
Rashes
Strengthens and tones the veins and the connective tissue of the blood vessels and skin.
Hemorrhoids and varicose veins.
3 times a day, add 15 drops in a small glass of water and drink in small sips.

Helleborus 3x
Overweight due to weak kidneys and a weak heart.
Stimulates the kidneys to extract metabolic waste and acid.
Strengthens the heart muscle.
3 times a day, take 10 globules, let them melt in the mouth.

Helonias dioica 3x
Overweight and connective tissue weakness of women.
Helonias strengthens the connective tissue of the skin.
Uterine prolapse
3 times a day, take 10 globules, let them melt in your mouth.

Hepatica triloba 3x
Overweight with high cholesterol and hyperlipidemia.
Stimulates the liver in cholesterol reduction and strengthens the pancreas in digestive functions.
Strengthens the pancreas, liver and spleen (the spleen is an important organ of defense).
3 times a day, take 10 globules, let them melt in your mouth.

Hypericum tincture
Overweight
Weight gain due to depression, nervousness and neurastenia.
A classic remedy for mental illness.
Affects mood enhancing, tonic and vegetative balancing.
3 times a day, add 15 drops in a small glass of water. Drink in small sips.

Iodine 12x (Jodum D12)
Overweight
An important remedy for the treatment of overweight due to a weak thyroid gland and pancreas.
Bloating, constipation and emaciation.
Hypothyroidism
The metabolism is stimulated and the immune system strengthened.
Diabetes
Arteriosclerosis (leading to an insufficient supply of oxygen and nutrients of the body cells).
2 times a day, take 5 globules, let them melt in your mouth.

Juglans cinerea 6x

Overweight with high cholesterol and hyperlipidemia due to disorders of pancreas and liver function.
Promotes bile formation. This supports fat metabolism. Stimulates the liver in cholesterol reduction and strengthens the pancreas in digestive functions.
3 times a day, take 5 globules, let them melt in your mouth.

Juniperus tincture

Overweight
Acidification and overload with toxins due to weak kidneys.
Purifies and detoxifies the body.
Purifying the organism and enhancing the immune system. Strengthens the kidneys and stomach.
Do not use in an acute kidney disease. Juniper tincture highly stimulates the kidneys.
2 times a day, add 10 drops in a small glass of water. Drink in small sips.

Kali carb 12x (Kalium carbonicum D12)
Overweight
The thyroid is underactive (causes weight gain)
Bad breath like cheese.
Weakness in the abdomen
After eating the symptoms are more worse.
General physical, mental and spiritual weakness.
Constant fear, fear of the future, of death. What should I do if .....
Tendency to cold
Stinging and wandering pain
Bags on the upper eyelids
Sweating at the slightest exertion
He is easily excited
Fear of being alone
A frightful man
Hypersensitivity to pain and noise
Bad memory, daytime sleepiness
2 times a day, take 5 globules, let them melt in your mouth.

Kalium jodatum 6x (Potassium iodatum D6)
Overweight due to an underactive thyroid gland and arterial circulatory disorders.
Kalium jodatum stimulates the thyroid gland.
Regulates blood vessel tension.
Promotes blood circulation (important for the treatment of weight gain).
A significant remedy to treat atherosclerosis.
Strengthens the immune system.
The patient seeks to relieve his discomfort in fresh air and wind.
Improvement in movement.
3 times a day, take 5 globules, let them melt in your mouth.

Lamii albi tincture
Overweight
Anemia and iron deficiency
Promotes the formation of blood.
3 times a day, add 15 drops in a small glass of water and drink in small sips.

Levisticum tincture
Overweight
Weight gain and edema due to cardiac and renal weakness.
Promotes blood circulation of the urogenital tract.
An aphrodisiac
3 times a day, add 15 drops in a small glass of water and drink in small sips.

Lilium tigrinum tincture
Overweight and connective tissue weakness of women in menopause.
Strengthens the skin, the walls of arteries and veins.
Women with menopausal symptoms, heart problems and circulatory problems.
Complaints by uterine prolapse in menopause.
Irritable mood states
3 times a day, add 15 drops in a small glass of water and drink in small sips.

Lithium carb 6x (Lithium carbonicum D6)
Overweight
To deacidify and detoxify the body.
Gout, rheumatic diseases.
Uric acid in the blood.
3 times a day, take 3 globules, let them melt in your mouth.

Lycopodium 6x
Overweight
Stops the nightly cravings and cravings for sweets.
Aggravation of symptoms between 4 pm and 8 pm, through heat, touch, anger and tight clothing.
Feeling of helplessness.
Complaints mostly on the right side of the body.
The typical "Lycopodium type" requires sweets, sugar and hot drinks.
He is nasty on awakening, but otherwise the symptoms are better in the morning.
Flatulence and bloating even after eating small amounts.
Irascibility, brooks no contradiction.
Disorders of pancreas and liver function.
Inflammation and disorders of the hepatobiliary system.
Swelling of the liver, obstinate constipation.
Sour vomiting
Flatulence and rumbling in the abdomen.
Much gas formation in the stomach, a loud rumbling and gurgling in the bowels.
Heartburn and great fatigue after eating.
Constant burping
Saturated after little food.
Improvement by belching, by hot food and drinks, exercise and cold air.
The pain is chronic and burning.
Kidney stones
Red gries (such as brick dust sediment) in the urine.
The "Lycopodium patient" has two strange symptoms:
"He weeps, if somebody would like to thank him" and "one foot is warm, the other foot is cold".
3 times a day, take 5 globules, let them melt in your mouth.

Madar 6x
Overweight
Affects the hunger center in the brain and curbs the appetite.
Detoxifying
3 times a day, take 5 globules, let them melt in your mouth.

Melilotus tincture
Overweight
Supports metabolism in the treatment of overweight.
Extracts metabolic waste and toxins.
Strengthens the immune system and supports the metabolism.
Weakness of the veins and lymphatic vessels.
Strengthens veins and lymphatic vessels.
Improves blood and lymph flow.
Thins the blood.
Strengthens the connective tissue.
Venous circulation disorders
Rush of blood to the head and red face.
Improvement through nosebleeds
3 times a day, add 15 drops in a small glass of water and drink in small sips.

Mercurius corossivus 6x
Overweight
Connective tissue weakness caused by degenerative blood vessels.
The skin is cold, pale and dripping with sweat.
Salivation with salty taste.
Weakness of memory
3 times a day, take 5 globules, let them melt in your mouth.

Mercurius dulcis 6x
Overweight
Diabetes
Promotes the secretion of the pancreas.
Inflammation of the liver-bile system.
Promotes bile flow
3 times a day, take 5 globules, let them melt in your mouth.

Millefolium tincture
Overweight
Relaxes and calms the entire abdomen.
Promotes the circulation of the digestive organs.
Bloating
Strengthens the spleen (important for the treatment of weight gain)
Promotes iron absorption in the small intestine.
Promotes blood circulation and strengthens the blood vessels. As a result, the body is better supplied with oxygen and nutrients and the metabolism will be strengthened.
Strengthens the immune system.
3 times a day, add 15 drops in a small glass of water and drink in small sips.

Myrtillus 3x
Weight gain
Stimulates in the treatment of overweight the detoxification of the body and metabolism.
Stimulates the detoxification through the skin.
Strengthens the pancreas.
Diabetes
3 times a day, take 10 globules, let them melt in your mouth.

Nasturtium officinale tincture
Overweight
Connective tissue weakness
Contains many important vitamins for the treatment of connective tissue weakness.
Chronic diseases
A natural antibiotic
3 times a day, add 15 drops in a small glass of water or in a cup of nettle tea. Drink in small sips.

Natrium choleinicum D6 (Sodium choleinicum D6)
Overweight
Metabolic disorders
Constipation and flatulence due to an insufficient bile production.
Promotes the secretion of the pancreas.
To increase the secretion of bile.
For the prevention of gallstones.
3 times a day, take 5 globules, let them melt in your mouth.

Nux vomica 6x

Overweight

Consequence of alcohol abuse, coffee, overeating and long nights.

High blood pressure due to stress and anger.

Overwrought nerves, nausea and vomiting.

Circulatory problems with vertigo, especially after stimulant abuse (alcohol, nicotine).

A feeling of constriction.

Tendency to convulsions and periodic complaints.

Diseases of the pancreas due to alcohol abuse.

Tearing, stinging and contractive pain in the abdomen.

Swelling of the liver

Gallstones

Inflammation of the bile ducts.

Large and hard stools. Always has the feeling that the evacuation would be incomplete.

Frequent need for toileting, but without success.

Feeling as if a stone in the stomach.

Frequent belching of sour or bitter liquid.

Fever

The "Nux vomica type":

Irritable, choleric, nervous, lively, emaciated.

He considers himself to be very important.

The Modalities:

Worse are the symptoms after midnight, in the early morning, by cold and dry weather, after drinking wine and coffee.

Improvement in wet weather, in warm rooms.

The pain: Tearing, astringent, cramping, dull.

3 times a day, take 5 globules, let them melt in your mouth.

Okoubaka

Weight gain and overweight

Toxins (for example food additives) block the metabolism. This causes acidification and overload with toxins. Okoubaka detoxifies the body, dissolves metabolic blockages, eliminates metabolic waste and environmental toxins.

Strengthens the immune system. Helps therefore good for the treatment of acidification and overload with toxins.

For thorough detoxification, elimination and excretion of environmental toxins and other residues, please make the following treatment. In addition, please drink the above mentioned teas.

1st to 4th week:
Okoubaka 3x
3 times a day, take 10 globules, let them melt in your mouth.

5th to 8th week:
Okoubaka 4x
3 times a day, take 10 globules, let them melt in your mouth.

9th to 12th week:
Okoubaka 6x
3 times a day, take 5 globules, let them melt in your mouth.

13th to 16th week:
Okoubaka 12x
2 times a day, take 5 globules, let them melt in your mouth.

Then a further 3 months:
Okoubaka 30x
1 time a week, take 5 globules, let them melt in your mouth.

Phaseolum tincture
Overweight
An excellent remedy to dissolve and eliminate water retentions in the body.
The main remedy for stimulating diuresis.
Proven in high uric acid and ascites (abdominal dropsy).
3 times a day, add 15 drops in a small glass of water and drink in small sips.

Phosphorus amorphus 12x
Overweight
Phosphorus is an important metabolic remedy for the treatment of weight gain.
Phosphorus strengthens the function of liver, pancreas and immune system.
Alternating diarrhea and constipation.
Craving for salt, cold drinks or ice cream.
Nervousness, hectic red spots on the face.
Nervous itching
Tingling or burning sensation between the shoulder blades.
A frosty person. Depression and self-pity.
Labile moods, he likes to be comforted.
Phosphorus is known in naturopathy as a "light bringer".
He is afraid of darkness, aloneness and thunderstorms.
Quickly furious. The patient reacts violently to everything.
The patient is exhausted quickly.
Night sweats
Scary, especially at dusk.
He is tall, blonde and has fine hair.
Bleed easily
Get bruises easily and is very sensitive to pain.
In rapid movements (turning the head) he get dizzy.
2 times a day, take 5 globules, let them melt in your mouth.

Podophyllum 6x
Weight gain
An important remedy for the treatment of overweight.
Constipation
Podophyllum stimulates the formation of juices in the pancreas and liver.
Disorders of the hepatobiliary system.
Gastritis and stomach ulcer.
Empty feeling in the stomach.
Morning sickness with vomiting.
Nausea and dizziness.
3 times a day, take 5 globules, let them melt in your mouth.

Psorinum 12x

Overweight

For the treatment of persistent metabolic disorders.

The typical "Psorinum patient" is frosty, cautious, afraid to wash and has an unpleasant perspiration.

Desperate anxiety

Chronic eczema and dermatitis.

Obstinate and itchy skin conditions

The skin is usually dry, pale and yellow.

Stinking foot sweat and stinking night sweats.

Lichen, scabs, acne and blackheads.

Aggravation from cold, sun, wind, and when changing from warm to cold weather.

Improvement by rest, when lying down and through eating.

2 times a day, take 5 globules, let them melt in your mouth.

Pulsatilla 6x
Overweight
Constipation after fat and a lot of food.
Diarrhea and constipation alternating.
Inflammation and disorders of the female reproductive organs.
Worse in a warmth, especially in warm rooms.
The "Pulsatilla Type" is moody, sensitive and whiny, loves compassion.
Lack of appetite, no thirst.
Neurasthenia and hypersensitivity to noise.
Self-pity
Moody, wants comfort, gentle, melancholy and anxious.
Has fear of death and is afraid of people.
Keynotes: Soft and gentle disposition, shy, timid, tearful, chilly, anemic.
3 times a day, take 5 globules, let them melt in your mouth.

Quassia amara 3x

Overweight due to a weakness of the pancreas and liver.
Cleanses the body fluids and stimulates the liver, gallbladder and pancreas.
Meteorism (Bloating)
An important metabolic remedy.
Strengthens the immune system.
Frontal headache (often a sign of liver dysfunction).
3 times a day, take 10 globules, let them melt in your mouth.

Rhizoma Helenii tincture

An excellent metabolic remedy for the treatment of overweight.
Strengthens and regenerates pancreas and liver.
Strengthens the immune system.
Diabetes
3 times a day, add 15 drops in a small glass of water and drink in small sips.

Rosmarinus tincture
Overweight
Stimulates the metabolism, blood circulation and the immune system.
Arterial circulatory disturbances.
Low blood pressure
Strengthens the heart and blood vessels.
Purifies and detoxifies the muscles and conective tissue.
This is important for the treatment of weight gain.
Very good for the treatment of rheumatism and metabolic acidosis.
3 times a day, add 15 drops in a small glass of water and drink in small sips.

Ruta graveolens 6x
Overweight
Arterial circulatory disorders
Rheumatism
Stimulates blood circulation and connective tissue.
Proven in rheumatic pain.
Muscle pain caused by overexertion
Inflamed muscles, ligaments and tendons
Tendovaginitis
In the morning the pain is worse.
Periosteum injuries
Worse by lying down.
The pain seems to come out from the bones.
The patient has to walk around to ease his pain.
3 times a day, take 5 globules, let them melt in your mouth.

Sanguinaria 6x
Weight gain of women in menopause.
Loss of smell and taste.
Hypersensitive to cold and weather changes, wind and "every change of clothes."
The symptoms appear and disappear with the sun.
Dizziness, depression and symptoms of menopause.
Meteorosensitivity with headache.
Burning of the hands and feet. Always red face.
3 times a day, take 5 globules, let them melt in your mouth.

Sepia 12x

Overweight in women.
Headache, sleeplessness, nervousness, depression and anxiety.
The woman sighs, moans and smiles alternately.
Dropping of the eyelids
Multiple disorders of the female reproductive organs.
Sad and cries often without knowing why.
The "Sepia type" has a yellowish complexion, hates compassion and wants to be left alone.
Mentally sluggish and irritable
Rapid change of mood
Indifferent to obligations
The stomach feels empty and desolate.
The hepatic region is painful and stinging.
Brown spots on the skin of the abdomen.
Diarrhea after milk consumption.
Feeling of heaviness in the rectum.
No relief after defecation
Pain in the rectum during defecation and long time after stool.
The stool is hard, knotty, too little, covered with blood and mucus.
2 times a day, take 5 globules, let them melt in your mouth.

Solidago tincture
Weight gain
Excretes during the treatment of overweight water retentions.
To stimulate the blood cleansing and extraction via the kidneys.
Diuretic
To stimulate the kidneys.
3 times a day, add 15 drops in a small glass of water or in a cup of nettle tea and drink in small sips.

Spongia 6x
Weight gain due to an underactive thyroid.
Stimulates the thyroid gland. The body temperature increases. The immune system and metabolism are strengthened.
3 times a day, take 5 globules, let them melt in your mouth.

Staphysagria 6x
Overweight
Staphysagria is a great remedy for suppressed anger and repressed emotions.
Agitation of mind and nervous system.
Great indignation about things that were done by others or himself.
Keynotes:
Sensitive to what others think about him.
Deep-set eyes with blue edges as after a night of drinking.
Modalities:
Worse at night, by anger and indignation.
Improvement of the symptoms after breakfast, by heat and bed rest.
3 times a day, take 5 globules, let them melt in your mouth.

Sulphur 12x

Weight gain due to a reduced metabolism.
Sulfur is an important catalyst to regenerate a sluggish and blocked metabolism.
The skin looks gray, dirty and wrinkled.
Itching and burning at night.
Stabbing pains in the liver.
Stinking flatulence in the morning.
Hunger at 11 clock in the morning (11 am).
Appetite for everything, especially on fat.
Pushes away the cover at night, stretching his legs out of bed.
Redness of the orifices.
Sharp and excoriating secretions.
Sulfur strengthens the immune system and regenerates the pancreas and liver.
Chronic diseases
Sulfur is detoxifying the body.
2 times a day, take 5 globules, let them melt in your mouth.

Symphytum 6x
Overweight
Wrinkles due to a weak connective tissue of the skin.
Strengthens the connective tissue and the metabolism.
Anemia and iron deficiency
Promotes the formation of blood.
Contains iron and vitamin B12.
Strengthens the spleen (important for the treatment of weight gain).
Promotes iron absorption in the small intestine.
Promotes hepatic blood flow and is important for the small intestine.
Strengthens the blood vessels.
3 times a day, take 5 globules, let them melt in your mouth.

Syzygium tincture
Overweight
Strengthens the function of pancreas, liver and gallbladder.
Proven in diabetes.
3 times a day, add 15 drops in a small glass of water and drink in small sips.

Taraxacum tincture (dandelion)
Weight gain due to weakness and diseases of the liver and bile.
Strengthens the liver-bile system, the pancreas and kidneys.
Detoxifies the liver and acts cholagogue.
Strengthens the immune system.
Cleans the blood and stimulates the metabolism.
Nausea due to a weakness of pancreas and liver.
3 times a day, add 15 drops in a small glass of water and drink in small sips.

Thuja 6x
Overweight
Immune deficiency
Thuja excretes toxins and strengthens the immune system.
Modalities:
Worse by cold, wet weather, change of weather, storm and tempest, after drinking tea and eating onions.
Improvement by heat, warm applications and re-emerging sweat.
The complaints are worse at 3 clock in the morning (3 am) and 15 clock in the afternoon (3 pm).
3 times a day, take 5 globules, let them melt in your mouth.

Urtica urens tincture
Overweight
Purifies and detoxifies the body.
Stimulates the kidneys and metabolism to extract acids, toxins and metabolic waste.
Itchy and inflamed skin rash with small pimples and blisters.
Diuretic
3 times a day, add 15 drops in a small glass of water and drink in small sips.

A homeopathic prescription for the treatment of overweight and for stimulating the metabolism:
Helianthus tuberosus 3x dil., Duboisia 3x dil., Euphorbia cyparissias 3x dil. aa 10.0, Extractum Fucus vesiculosus (if not overactive thyroid occurs), Extractum Frangulae (buckthorn bark), Extractum Alchemilla (Lady's Mantle) aa 15.0
3 times a day, add 15 drops in a small glass of water and drink in small sips before eating.

A recipe in weight gain for strengthening the pancreas, liver and bile:
Cardui marianae tincture, Cardui Benedikti tincture aa 25.0, China tincture, Chelidonium tincture aa 10.0, Flor de Piedra 6x 30.0
3 times a day, add 15 drops in a small glass of water and drink in small sips.

Homeopathic recipes to treat overweight due to circulatory disorders.

1) Homeopathic prescription to treat overweight due to arteriosclerosis:
Arnica 3x, Potassium iodatum 6x (Kalium jodatum D6) aa 25.0
3 times a day, add 15 drops in a small glass of water and drink in small sips.

2) In general circulatory disorders:
Arnica tincture, Secale cornutum 6x aa 10.0, Tincture of Gingko biloba ad 50.0
3 times a day, add 15 drops in a small glass of water and drink in small sips.

3) Sanicula tincture, Millefolium tincture aa 50.0
3 times a day, add 15 drops in a small glass of water and drink in small sips.

4) Overweight due to arteriosclerosis and circulatory problems of women in menopause:
Secale cornutum 6x 10.0, Potassium iodatum 6x (Kalium jodatum D6) 10.0, Cimicifuga 6x 10.0
3 times a day, add 15 drops in a small glass of water and drink in small sips.

5) Overweight with circulatory disorders of the coronary arteries:
Potassium iodatum 4x (potassium is very important for the function of the heart muscle), Arnica tincture (vasodilator), Cactus grandiflorus 3x aa 10.0, Extractum Crataegi 20.0
3 times a day, add 15 drops in a small glass of water and drink in small sips.

Also homeopathic remedies for the lymph system are important for the treatment and prevention of weight gain and overweight. These remedies stimulate the excretion of acids, metabolic waste and toxins. They also purify and strengthen the function of the connective tissue and stimulate the immune system.

Therefore you also should take one of the following remedies:

1) Badiaga 12x
For 4 weeks, 2 times a day, take 5 globules. Let them melt in your mouth.

2) Baryta carbonica 12x (Barium carbonicum D12)
For 4 weeks, 2 times a day, take 5 globules. Let them melt in your mouth.

3) Barium iodatum 12x (Barium jodatum D12)
For 4 weeks, 2 times a day, take 5 globules. Let them melt in your mouth.

4) Calcarea 12x (Calcium carbonicum D12)
For 4 weeks, 2 times a day, take 5 globules. Let them melt in your mouth.

5) Mercury solubilis 12x (Mercurius solubilis D12)
For 4 weeks, 2 times a day, take 5 globules. Let them melt in your mouth.

6) Thuja 12x
For 4 weeks, 2 times a day, take 5 globules. Let them melt in your mouth.

Lose weight and stay slim with Schuessler salts

Now I will give you recommendations for weight loss and how to treat your overweight with the help of Schuessler salts (Biochemistry) and to activate your metabolism.

Weight gain can also be caused and reinforced by a mineral deficiency, because mineral deficiency weaken the metabolism and the immune system. The use of Schuessler salts (also named Biochemistry, cell salts, tissue salts) is a good way to compensate this mineral deficiency in a natural way.

A defective metabolism favors overweight, a weak immune system and health problems, and is often the result of a disturbance of mineral distribution and mineral intake. Although we may receive enough minerals in our food, in the event of a metabolic disorder, not all of the minerals may reach the cells.

Deficiency of mineral salts weaken the immune system, disrupt the hormonal balance and slow down the metabolism. Mineral salt deficiency can trigger cravings because the body tries to compensate the deficiency in the cells.

Stress, acidification of the body as well as environmental toxins hinder the mineral transport through the cell membranes. This is where the effect of biochemistry (Schuessler salts, cell salts) works. Biochemistry activates the excretion of toxins and acids. The organism is purified from inside.

The result: The basal metabolic rate increases, more energy is consumed, the body breaks down fat reserves.

Prerequisite to avoid and to treat overweight is a balanced acid-base-balance, proper nutrition and good blood circulation. Nutrition is a key factor in the treatment of our metabolism and health. With a balanced and varied diet the body will be supplied with all the necessary nutrients. The cells and organs are strengthened.

At the same time you support your immune system, your metabolism and ensure a perfect acid-base-balance, the foundation of our health. Proper nutrition also helps to excrete toxins from the body and dissolves healing blockages.

Remember: There are several metabolic blockages which you have to treat for to deacidify and detoxify the body of people suffering from weight gain and overweight.

Metabolic blockage No. 1: The acid-base balance

Too much sugar, white flour, meat and sausage acidifies the body. In order to neutralize the acids precious bases are consumed. What is not neutralized, ends up as a "hazardous waste" in the connective tissue and leads to its acidity.

The metabolic process slows down. We gain weight despite calorie conscious diet and exercise.

Schuessler-salt No. 9 Sodium phosphate D6 (Nr. 9 Natrium phosphoricum D6) ensures that toxins and metabolic residues are flushed from the body. Sodium phosphate (Natrium phosphoricum) also stimulates the metabolism of fat and sugar degradation.

Metabolic blockage No. 2: The connective tissue

The connective tissue is more than just a connection between the organs. It serves as a nutrient storage and intermediate storage of metabolic products. In the connective tissue the cells dispose their waste products. That the toxins can leave the body, enough mineral salts must be present.

A mineral deficiency causes metabolic residues, acidification and overload with toxins. They remain in the connective tissue and bind water. It comes to overweight and water retention (edema) in the tissues of the body.

The salts No. 6 Potassium sulph D6 (Nr. 6 Kalium sulfuricum D6), No. 9 Sodium phosphate D6 (Nr. 9 Natrium phosphoricum D6), No. 10 Sodium sulphate D6 (Nr. 10 Natrium sulfuricum D6) and No. 11 Silicea D12 promote the excretion of acids and toxins through the skin and activate the detoxification via the liver, intestines and kidneys.

Metabolic blockage No. 3: The digestion

Environmental pollution, lush diet and medication burden the liver, our central metabolic organ. Stomach, pancreas and intestines suffer with. Many metabolic processes stalled and it comes to weight gain, constipation, bloating and stomach problems.

No. 4 Potassium chloratum D6 (Nr. 4 Kalium chloratum D6), No. 6 Potassium sulph D6 (Nr. 6 Kalium sulfuricum D6) and No. 10 Sodium sulphate (Nr. 10 Natrium sulfuricum D6) give the liver and digestive organs new power. The metabolic processes accelerate. Toxins and acids are excreted faster.

Metabolic blockage No. 4: Our water Resources

Every day the organism produces acids and waste products that have to be filtered out by the kidneys. But part of it also ends up in the connective tissue, because for the removal mineral salts are absent. We gain weight.

No. 8 Sodium chloratum D6 (Nr. 8 Natrium chloratum D6) regulates the water balance and No. 10 Sodium sulphate D6 (Nr. 10 Natrium sulfuricum D6) drained. Together they controll the water balance in the body.

Metabolic blockage No. 5: The protein digestion

Protein is essential for the production of enzymes, hormones, muscles and the connective tissue. However, in the cleavage of proteins ammonia is formed (a strong cytotoxin). The liver converts the ammonia into non-toxic urea, which is excreted in the urine.

Therefore, a high intake of protein is a strong decontamination work for the liver and our two kidneys. The result is overweight.

Salt No. 9 Sodium phosphate D6 (Nr. 9 Natrium phosphoricum D6) helps the body in protein metabolism. Salt No. 6 Potassium sulph D6 (Nr. 6 Kalium sulfuricum D6) supports the liver in the degradation of ammonia.

Metabolic blockage No. 6: The digestion of fat

We need fats because they provide essential fatty acids. But fat is also the best energy storage in times of need. The body hoards it especially in the thighs and hips, the abdomen and buttocks.

But the adipose tissue is also a deposit for toxins and forces weight gain.

The Schuessler salts No. 6 Potassium sulph D6 (Nr. 6 Kalium sulfuricum D6), No. 9 Sodium phosphate D6 (Nr. 9 Natrium phosphoricum D6) and No. 10 Sodium sulphate D6 (Nr. 10 Natrium sulfuricum D6) help to lead out the contaminants.

Metabolic blockage No. 7: The carbohydrate digestion

Carbohydrates are energy pure. But in abundance they are also responsible for weight gain and acidification of the body. What is not burned, will be converted and stored in fat.

Especially sweets and white flour products are dangerous. They let the blood sugar level rise up rapidly. This leads to a strong insulin release.

Insulin normalizes blood sugar. At the same time burning fat is broken. Insulin leads fats from the meal into the fat stores of the body. In addition, it holds back water in the body and causes rapidly new hunger.

The Schuessler salt No. 4 Potassium chloratum D6 (Nr. 4 Kalium chloratum D6) supports the combustion of sugar. Important are also the salts No. 6 Potassium sulph D6 (Nr. 6 Kalium sulphuricum D6) and No. 10 Sodium sulphate D6 (Nr 10 Natrium sulfuricum D6).

The combination of these salts Nos. 4, 6, 8, 9, 10 and 11 has proven itself well in the treatment of acidification and overload with toxins. Dissolve from each cell salt 1 tablet in a small glass of hot water (all together in the same glass). Drink in small sips half an hour before or after eating.

After 6 weeks you make one week break, then repeat. If necessary, you can repeat this treatment several times.

Hunger is the enemy of all weight loss attempts:

Against continuous hunger:
No. 6 Potassium sulph 6x (Nr. 6 Kalium sulfuricum D6) and
No. 10 Sodium sulphate 6x (Nr. 10 Natrium sulfuricum D6)
Alternate each remedy hourly by taking 4 times a day 2 tablets. Let them melt in your mouth.

Desire for sweets:
No. 7 Magnesium phophate 6x (Nr. 7 Magnesium phosphoricum D6) and
No. 9 Sodium phosphate 6x (Nr. 9 Natrium phosphoricum D6)
Alternate each remedy half-hourly by taking 2 tablets. Let them melt in your mouth.

Craving for fat:
No. 5 Potassium phosphate 6x (Nr. 5 Kalium phosphoricum D6) and
No. 9 Sodium phosphate 6x (Nr. 9 Natrium phosphoricum D6)
Alternate each remedy half-hourly by taking 2 tablets. Let them melt in your mouth.

Craving for chocolate:
No. 7 Magnesium phosphate 6x (Nr. 7 Magnesium phosphoricum D6)
Half-hourly take 2 tablets. Let them melt in your mouth.

Craving for salty food:
No. 8 Sodium chloratum 6x (Nr. 8 Natrium chloratum D6)
Half-hourly take 2 tablets. Let them melt in your mouth.

Craving for bitter and hearty food:
No. 10 Sodium sulphate 6x (Nr. 10 Natrium sulfuricum D6)
Half-hourly take 2 tablets. Let them melt in your mouth.

Craving for nuts:
No. 5 Potassium phosphate 6x (Nr. 5 Kalium phosphoricum D6)
Half-hourly take 2 tablets. Let them melt in your mouth.

Craving for sour food:
No. 9 Sodium phosphate 6x (Nr. 9 Natrium phosphoricum D6)
Half-hourly take 2 tablets. Let them melt in your mouth.

Weight loss with Homeopathy and Schuessler salts

Biochemical health cure (Schuessler salts) for losing weight: The following cell salts are proven in the treatment of obesity in conjunction with a calorie conscious diet and physical activity.
Duration: 6 weeks, then 1 week off. If necessary, repeat several times.

No. 4 Potassium chloratum 6x (Nr. 4 Kalium chloratum D6) [5]
No. 9 Sodium phosphate 6x (Nr. 9 Natrium phosphoricum D6) and [10]
No. 10 Sodium sulphate 6x (Nr. 10 Natrium sulfuricum D6) [11]
Alternate each remedy daily by taking 4 times a day 2 tablets. Let them melt in your mouth.

Helios Nos:

The above mentioned cell salts have the following effects:
1) No. 4 Potassium chloratum 6x (Nr. 4 Kalium chloratum D6) [5]
- Reduces fat and overweight.
- Relieves cravings
  Helps eliminate toxins
  Directs waste materials out of the body
  Strengthens the circulation
  Helps to prevent the listlessness

2) No. 9 Sodium phosphate 6x (Nr. 9 Natrium phosphoat D6)
- Reduces fat and overweight.
- Relieves cravings for sweets and fat food.
Regulates the acid-base-balance. This relieves the metabolism and cholesterol is excreted faster. Increased blood lipid levels will be reduced.
Effective against atherosclerosis
Helps against cellulite
Makes you thirsty for water
Has a normalizing effect on the gastrointestinal tract.

3) No. 10 Sodium sulphate 6x (Nr. 10 Natrium sulfuricum D6)
- Reduces overweight and fat
- Relieves cravings
Promotes the fat metabolism
Stimulating the metabolism
Reduces toxins
Strengthens the blood circulation
Helps against cellulite and edema
Strengthens the digestive system
Makes you thirsty for water
Promotes bile formation in the liver. The cholesterol is thereby broken down and excreted faster.
Hepatobiliary disorders
Stimulates the excretion of metabolic waste via the liver, gallbladder and kidneys.
Strengthens the pancreas, liver, gallbladder and kidneys.

A proven biochemical treatment for detoxification, purification and stimulation of metabolism (important for weight loss and the treatment of overweight): Duration: 6 weeks, then 1 week off. Repeat 2 times. Make at the same time a low-calorie diet and adequate exercise.

No. 1 Calcium fluorite 12x (Nr. 1 Calcium fluoratum D12)
No. 3 Ferrum phos 12x (Nr. 3 Ferrum phosphoricum D12)
No. 8 Sodium chloratum 6x (Nr. 8 Natrium chloratum D6)
No. 9 Sodium phosphate 6x (Nr. 9 Natrium phosphoricum D6)
No. 4 Potassium chloratum 6x (Nr. 4 Kalium chloratum D6)
No. 10 Sodium sulphate 6x (Nr. 10 Natrium sulfuricum D6) and
No. 6 Potassium sulph 6x (Nr. 6 Kalium sulphuricum D6)
Alternate each remedy daily by taking 4 times a day 2 tablets. Let them melt in your mouth.

In addition take every evening:
No. 11 Silicea 12x
Increases the strength and resistance of the connective tissue, promotes the function of the lymphatic system. From 4 pm 3 times take 2 tablets. Let them melt in your mouth.

More Schuessler salts (Biochemistry) for losing weight and for the treatment and prevention of overweight, weight gain and obesity:

Too much body weight with elevated cholesterol level, to stimulate bile formation:
No. 20 Potassium aluminum sulph 6x (Nr. 20 Kalium aluminium sulfuricum D6) and
No. 7 Magnesium phosphate 6x
Alternate each remedy daily by taking 4 times a day 2 tablets. Let them melt in your mouth.

Too much body weight and acidification of the body:
No. 11 Silicea 12x and
No. 9 Sodium phosphate 6x (Nr. 9 Natrium phosphoricum D6)
Alternate each remedy daily by taking 4 times a day 2 tablets. Let them melt in your mouth.

Too much body weight, elevated cholesterol level, to improve the function of the liver:
No. 7 Magnesium phosphate 6x (Nr. 7 Magnesium phosphoricum D6)
No. 10 Sodium sulphate 6x (Nr. 10 Natrium sulfuricum D6) and
No. 11 Silicea 12x
Alternate each remedy daily by taking 4 times a day 2 tablets. Let them melt in your mouth.

If the skin feels spongy and flabby:
No. 2 Calcium phosphate 6x (Nr. 2 Calcium phosphoricum D6)
No. 8 Sodium chloratum 6x (Nr. 8 Natrium chloratum D6) and
No. 10 Sodium sulph 6x (Nr. 10 Natrium sulfuricum D6)
Alternate each remedy daily by taking 4 times a day 2 tablets. Let them melt in your mouth.

Overweight with liver disease and a bitter taste in the mouth:
No. 10 Sodium sulphate 6x (Nr. 10 Natrium sulfuricum D6)
4 times a day, take 2 tablets. Let them melt in your mouth.

To stimulate the kidneys (important for the treatment of overweight):
No. 10 Sodium sulph 6x (Nr. 10 Natrium sulfuricum D6) and
No. 8 Sodium chloratum 6x (Nr. 8 Natrium chloratum D6)
Strengthen the kidneys to extract waste products.
Alternate each remedy daily by taking 4 times a day 2 tablets. Let them melt in your mouth.

Too much body weight with hemorrhoids:
No. 1 Calcium fluorite 12x (Nr. 1 Calcium fluoratum D12)
No. 9 Sodium phosphate 6x (Nr. 9 Natrium phosphat D6)
and
No. 10 Sodium sulphate 6x (Nr. 10 Natrium sulfuricum D6)
Alternate each remedy daily by taking 4 times a day 2 tablets. Let them melt in your mouth.

Overweigh with fatty degeneration of the heart muscle:
No. 1 Calcium fluorite 12x (Nr. 1 Calcium fluoratum D12)
and
No. 5 Potassium phosphate 6x (Nr. 5 Kalium phosphoricum D6)
Alternate each remedy daily by taking 4 times a day 2 tablets. Let them melt in your mouth.

Overweight with nervous debility and exhaustion:

1) Restlessness, nervousness and aggression:
No. 9 Sodium phosphate 6x (Nr. 9 Natrium phosphoricum D6) and
No. 16 Lithium chloratum 3x
Alternate each remedy daily by taking 4 times a day 2 tablets. Let them melt in your mouth.

2) Nervousness, emptiness and hollowness in the head, weakness:
No. 5 Potassium phosphate 6x (Nr. 5 Kalium phosphoricum D6)
No. 7 Magnesium phosphate 6x (Nr. 7 Magnesium phosphoricum D6) and
No. 8 Sodium chloratum 6x (Nr. 8 Natrium chloratum D6)
Alternate each remedy daily by taking 4 times a day 2 tablets. Let them melt in your mouth.

3) Nerve weakness, anemia and general debility (promotes obesity):
No. 2 Calcium phosphate 6x (Nr. 2 Calcium phosphoricum D6) and
No. 8 Sodium chloratum 6x (Nr. 8 Natrium chloratum D6)
Alternate each remedy daily by taking 4 times a day 2 tablets. Let them melt in your mouth.

4) General nervousness:
No. 7 Magnesium phosphate 6x (Nr. 7 Magnesium phosphoricum D6) and
No. 5 Potassium phosphate 6x (Nr. 5 Kalium phosphoricum D6)
The nutrient salt for body, mind, spirit and heart.
Promotes recovery and reconstruction.
Excitation and exhaustion of body and mind.
Brings the nerves metabolism back into balance.
Alternate each remedy daily by taking 4 times a day 2 tablets. Let them melt in your mouth.

To force the excretion of environmental toxins (cause cell blockade, obesity and a weakening of the immune system):
No. 8 Sodium phosphate 3x (Nr. 8 Natrium phosphoricum D3)
No. 2 Calcium phosphate 6x (Nr. 2 Calcium phosphoricum D6) and
No. 11 Silicea 12x
Alternate each remedy daily by taking 4 times a day 2 tablets. Let them melt in your mouth.

Biochemical health cure (Schuessler salts) for the treatment of overweight and weight gain because of an acidification of the body. The symptoms are rheumatism, gout, acid sweat, heartburn and acid regurgitation. Take 2 months in daily exchange:

1) No. 1 Calcium fluorite 12x (Nr. 1 Calcium fluoratum D12)
4 times a day, take 2 tablets, let them melt in your mouth.

2) No. 11 Silicea 12x
4 times a day, take 2 tablets, let them melt in your mouth.

3) No. 7 Magnesium phosphate 6x (Nr. 7 Magnesium phosphoricum D6)
4 times a day, take 2 tablets, let them melt in your mouth.

4) No. 9 Sodium phosphate 6x (Nr. 9 Natrium phosphoricum D6)
4 times a day, take 2 tablets, let them melt in your mouth.

Biochemical health cure for the regeneration of the pancreas (very important for weight loss):

1) No. 4 Potassium chloratum 6x (Nr. 4 Kalium chloratum D6)
The main means of all glands.
4 times a day, 2 tablets, let them melt in your mouth.
Alternating daily with the homeopathic remedy
Magnesium fluorite 6x (optimizes the effect of Potassium chloratum).
4 times a day, take 2 tablets, let them melt in your mouth.

After 3 weeks take for 2 weeks:
No. 6 Potassium sulph 6x (Nr. 6 Kalium sulphuricum D6)
alternating daily with
No. 10 Sodium sulphate 6x (Nr. 10 Natrium sulphuricum D6)
4 times a day, take 2 tablets, let them melt in your mouth.

External biochemical applications:

Schuessler ointment No. 1 Calcium fluorite (Nr. 1 Calcium fluoratum) alternating daily with ointment No. 11 Silica and No. 6 Potassium sulph (Nr. 6 Kalium sulfuricum):
Strengthens the skin and connective tissue. The skin gets more tensional force in order to adapt to the body becoming slimmer.
Calcium fluorite helps combat sagging tissue, wrinkles and hardening of the tissue.

Biochemical treatment to stimulate blood circulation and to force the metabolism (both are important in the treatment of too much body weight). Duration of intake: 2 months

On Monday
No. 1 Calcium fluorite 12x (Nr. 1 Calcium fluoratum D12)
4 times a day, take 2 tablets, let them melt in your mouth.

On Tuesday
No. 3 Ferrum phos 6x (Nr. 3 Ferrum phosphoricum D12)
4 times a day, take 2 tablets, let them melt in your mouth.

On Wednesday
No. 5 Potassium phosphate 6x (Nr. 5 Kalium phosphoricum D6)
4 times a day, take 2 tablets, let them melt in your mouth.

On Thursday
No. 1 Calcium fluorite 12x
4 times a day, take 2 tablets, let them melt in your mouth.

On Friday
No. 7 Magnesium phosphate 6x (Nr. 7 Magnesium phosphoricum D6)
4 times a day, take 2 tablets, let them melt in your mouth.

On Saturday
No. 1 Calcium fluorite 12x
4 times a day, take 2 tablets, let them melt in your mouth.

On Sunday
No. 3 Ferrum phos 12x
4 times a day, take 2 tablets, let them melt in your mouth.

Biochemical health cure (Schuessler salts) for the treatment of weight gain and for strengthening the connective tissue, veins and arteries. Duration of intake: 2 months

On Monday
No. 1 Calcium fluorite 12x (Nr. 1 Calcium fluoricum D12)
4 times a day, take 2 tablets, let them melt in your mouth.

On Tuesday
No. 11 Silicea 12x
4 times a day, take 2 tablets, let them melt in your mouth.

On Wednesday
No. 9 Sodium phosphate 6x (Nr. 9 Natrium phosphoricum D6)
4 times a day, take 2 tablets, let them melt in your mouth.

On Thursday
No. 1 Calcium fluorite 12x
4 times a day, take 2 tablets, let them melt in your mouth.

On Friday
No. 11 Silicea 12x
4 times a day, take 2 tablets, let them melt in your mouth.

On Saturday
No. 1 Calcium fluorite 12x (Nr. 1 Calcium fluoratum D12)
4 times a day, take 2 tablets, let them melt in your mouth.

On Sunday
No. 9 Sodium phosphate 6x
4 times a day, take 2 tablets, let them melt in your mouth.

Biochemical health cure (Schuessler salts) to treat overweight, neurasthenia, anxiety and irritability. Duration: 2 months

Monday
No. 7 Magnesium phosphate 6x
4 times a day, take 2 tablets, let them melt in your mouth.

Tuesday
No. 5 Potassium phosphate 6x (Nr. 5 Kalium ohosphoricum D6)
4 times a day, take 2 tablets, let them melt in your mouth.

Wednesday
No. 7 Magnesium phosphate 6x
4 times a day, take 2 tablets, let them melt in your mouth.

Thursday
No. 3 Ferrum phos 12x
4 times a day, take 2 tablets, let them melt in your mouth.

Friday
No. 7 Magnesium phosphate 6x
4 times a day, take 2 tablets, let them melt in your mouth.

Saturday
No. 5 Potassium phosphate 6x (Nr. 5 Kalium phosphoricum D6)
4 times a day, take 2 tablets, let them melt in your mouth.

Sunday
No. 3 Ferrum phos 12x
4 times a day, 2 tablets, let them melt in your mouth.

Biochemical health cure (Schuessler salts) for the treatment of overweight with liver and gallbladder disease, with bitter taste in the mouth, vomiting and sensitivity to changes in weather. Duration: 2 months

Monday
No. 7 Magnesium phosphate 6x (Nr. 7 Magnesium phosphoricum D6)
4 times a day, take 2 tablets, let them melt in your mouth.

Tuesday
No. 10 Sodium sulphate 6x (Nr. 10 Natrium sulfuricum D6)
4 times a day, take 2 tablets, let them melt in your mouth.

Wednesday
No. 7 Magnesium phosphate 6x
4 times a day, take 2 tablets, let them melt in your mouth.

Thursday
No. 6 Potassium sulph 6x (Nr. 6 Kalium sulfuricum D6)
4 times a day, take 2 tablets, let them melt in your mouth.

Friday
No. 7 Magnesium phosphate 6x
4 times a day, take 2 tablets, let them melt in your mouth.

Saturday
No. 10 Sodium sulphate 6x
4 times a day, take 2 tablets, let them melt in your mouth.

Sunday
No. 6 Potassium sulph 6x
4 times a day, take 2 tablets, let them melt in your mouth.

A biochemical health cure (Schuessler salts) to treat overweight and circulatory disorders. Duration: 2 months

Monday
No. 1 Calcium fluorite 12x (Nr. 1 Calcium fluoratum D12)
4 times a day, take 2 tablets, let them melt in your mouth.

Tuesday
No. 2 Calcium phosphate 6x (Nr. 2 Calcium phosphoricum D6)
4 times a day, take 2 tablets, let them melt in your mouth.

Wednesday
Nr. 11 Silicea 12x
4 times a day, take 2 tablets, let them melt in your mouth.

Thursday
No. 3 Ferrum phos 12x (Nr. 3 Ferrum phosphoricum D12)
4 times a day, take 2 tablets, let them melt in your mouth.

Friday
No. 7 Magnesium phosphate 6x (Nr. 7 Magnesium phosphoricum D6)
4 times a day, take 2 tablets, let them melt in your mouth.

Saturday
No. 1 Calcium fluorite 12x
4 times a day, take 2 tablets, let them melt in your mouth.

Sunday
No. 2 Calcium phosphate 6x
4 times a day, take 2 tablets, let them melt in your mouth.

More information about Schuessler salts you will find in my book:

Schuessler Salts - Homeopathic cell salts for your health

Epilogue

I hope that you have discovered a lot of new and interesting things while reading this book.

I wish you much success in the treatment and prevention of overweight and weight gain with Homeopathy and Schuessler salts, and wish you joy in life and especially your health.

Robert Kopf

Printed in Great Britain
by Amazon